NUTRITION

FOR

LIFE LONG WELLNESS

A Comprehensive Guide to Eating for Health and Healing

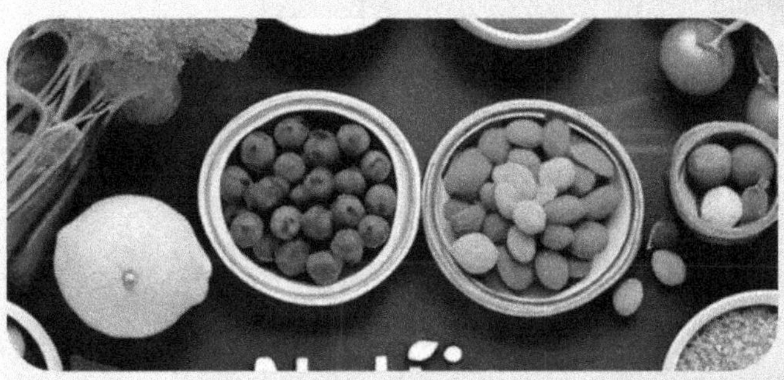

Dr J. B. TERRY

FIRST EDITION OCT. 2023

TABLE OF CONTENTS

INTRODUCTION

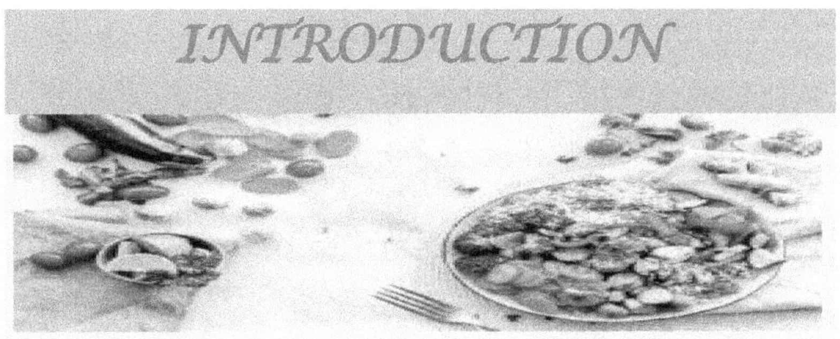

Welcome to "Nutrition for Lifelong Wellness: Achieve Vibrant Health with Balanced Nutrition." In this book, we'll explore how balanced nutrition can profoundly impact your lifelong well-being.

Your food choices go beyond satisfying hunger; they nurture your body and mind, support your health, and enhance your quality of life. We'll dive into the seven classes of food, revealing their roles in your overall health, and guide you in creating balanced meals that provide essential nutrients.

This journey is not just about the foods you eat. It's also about understanding the emotional aspects of eating, the link between nutrition and exercise, and the factors influencing your dietary choices.

As we progress, you'll learn to personalize your nutrition plan, whether you're in your youth, adulthood, or golden years. We'll explore dietary choices for special needs, including vegetarian, vegan, and plant-based diets, and offer practical guidance and recipes.

You'll leave with a personalized, practical, and balanced nutrition plan. This book equips you with the knowledge and tools to achieve your health and wellness goals, whether it's weight management, building strength, preventing illness, or simply leading a healthier life.

Thank you very much for joining us on this enlightening journey. Let's begin.

CHAPTER 1

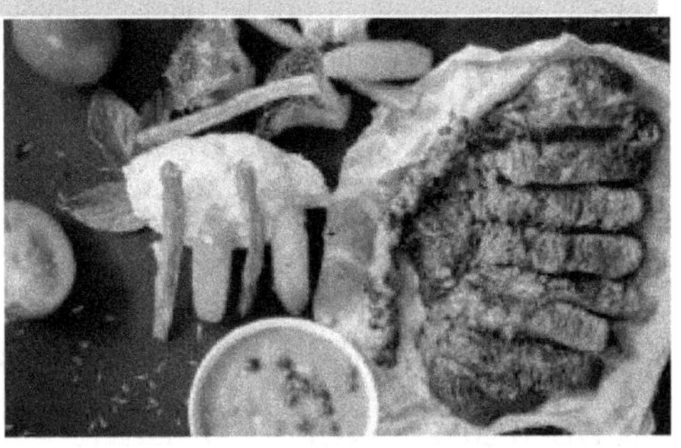

In our journey toward better health and healing through nutrition, it's crucial to start with a fundamental understanding of the seven essential classes of food. These seven categories form the building blocks of our diet and provide the nutrients our bodies need to thrive. Let's explore each of them:

1. **Carbohydrates:** Carbohydrates are the body's major source of energy. They come in two main forms: simple (sugars) and complex (starches and fiber). Simple carbs, found in foods like fruits and sweets, provide quick energy, while complex carbs, found in grains,

legumes, and vegetables, offer sustained energy and essential fiber for digestion.

2. Proteins: Proteins are the body's building blocks, essential for growth, repair, and maintaining body tissues. Meat, poultry, fish, eggs, dairy, legumes, and nuts are examples of sources of protein. A variety of protein sources ensures a diverse amino acid profile, supporting overall health.

3. Fats: Dietary fats serve various roles, from energy storage to insulation and protecting vital organs. Healthy fats, such as those found in avocados, nuts, and olive oil, support heart health and overall well-being. It's essential to balance saturated and trans fats, often found in processed and fried foods, to promote good health.

4. Vitamins: Vitamins are organic compounds that your body needs in small amounts for various functions. They play a critical role in immune function, metabolism, and overall health. Vitamins are typically obtained from a balanced diet that includes a variety of fruits, vegetables, and whole grains.

5. Minerals: Minerals are inorganic substances required for various physiological processes, including bone health, nerve function, and maintaining electrolyte balance. Key minerals include calcium, magnesium, and potassium. These can be found in dairy products, leafy greens, and bananas.

6. Fiber: Fiber is a type of carbohydrate that the body can't digest but is vital for digestive health. It aids in regulating blood sugar, reducing cholesterol levels, and maintaining a healthy weight. Perfect sources of fiber include the following: whole grains, fruits, vegetables, and legumes.

7. Water: Water is often overlooked but is perhaps the most critical nutrient. It makes up a significant portion of our bodies and is essential for all bodily functions, from digestion to temperature regulation. Staying well-hydrated is crucial for overall health and energy.

Understanding the role of these seven classes of food is the first step toward making informed dietary choices that promote health and healing. In the chapters that follow, we'll delve deeper into how to balance and optimize these nutrients to create a diet tailored to your specific needs and goals.

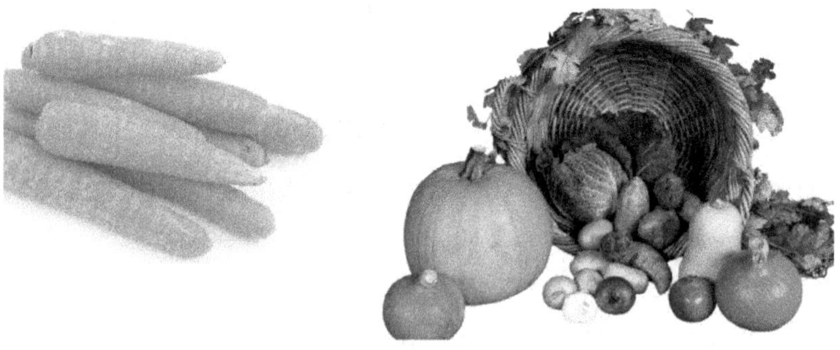

CHAPTER 2

THE IMPORTANCE OF BALANCE

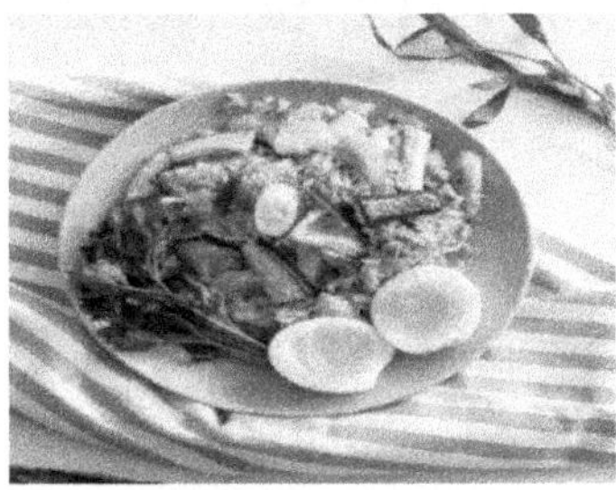

A well-balanced diet is the cornerstone of good health and healing. It's not just about what you eat but how you combine these essential classes of food to provide your body with the nutrients it needs. Let's explore the significance of balance in your diet and why it's vital for your overall well-being.

1. Nutrient Harmony:

- Imagine your body as a symphony of nutrients. Each class of food plays a unique instrument in this orchestra. Carbohydrates provide energy, proteins build and repair, fats support bodily functions, vitamins and minerals act as conductors, and fiber ensures smooth coordination. A balanced diet ensures that this symphony plays harmoniously.

2. Energy Balance:

- Carbohydrates supply the primary source of energy. Consuming too many can lead to excess calories and potential weight gain. On the other hand, not getting enough can leave you fatigued. Finding the right balance is essential for sustained energy levels throughout the day.

3. Protein for Tissue Repair:

- Proteins are vital for repairing and building tissues. A balanced intake ensures that your body has the necessary amino acids to maintain and renew muscles, skin, and organs. Consuming too little protein can lead to muscle weakness and slow recovery from illnesses.

4. Healthy Fats for Vital Functions:

- Fats are essential for vital functions like absorbing fat-soluble vitamins and maintaining healthy cell membranes. A balanced approach ensures you get the benefits without the risks of excess saturated and trans fats, which can harm your cardiovascular system.

5. Vitamins and Minerals for Health:

- Vitamins and minerals play specific roles in maintaining your health. Balance in this context means having a diet that provides all the necessary micronutrients in the right amounts. Deficiency or excess of any vitamin or mineral can lead to health issues.

6. Fiber for Digestive Health:

- A balanced diet implies an adequate intake of dietary fiber. Fiber aids in promoting healthy digestion, it also prevents constipation, and equally aids in weight management. Too little fiber can lead to digestive discomfort and other health problems.

7. Hydration for Well-Being:

- Water, often overlooked as a nutrient, is the ultimate balancer. It ultimately regulates body temperature, also transports nutrients, and removes waste. Maintaining a balanced state of hydration is fundamental for optimal bodily functions.

In this chapter, we've emphasized the importance of balance in your diet. It's not about excluding any of the seven classes of food but rather about consuming them in the right proportions. A well-balanced diet not only supports health and healing but also helps prevent a range of diet-related health problems.

CHAPTER 3

The timing of your meals can significantly impact your health and overall 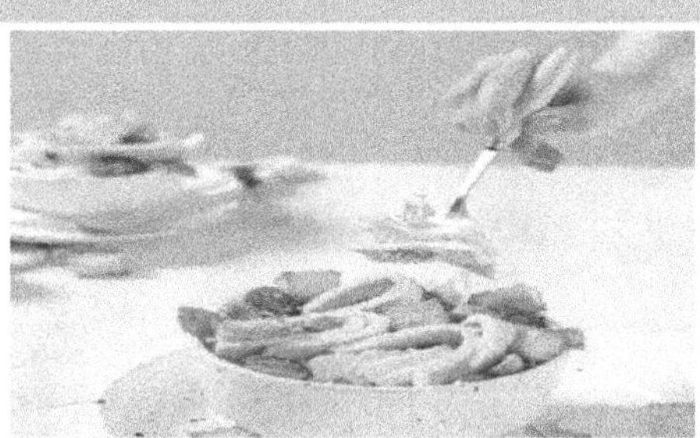 *well-being. In this chapter, we'll explore the importance of when to eat and how to structure your daily meals for optimal health and healing.*

1. Breakfast: The Foundation of Your Day:

- **<u>Breakfast is rightly considered the most essential meal of the day.</u>** After hours of fasting during sleep, your body needs fuel to kickstart your metabolism and provide energy for the day ahead. A balanced breakfast rich in complex carbohydrates, protein, and healthy fats can set a positive tone for your day.

2. Mid-Morning Snack: Sustaining Energy:

- Around mid-morning, a small, nutritious snack can maintain your energy levels and prevent overeating at lunch. Choose foods like yogurt, fruit, or nuts to keep your blood sugar stable.

3. Lunch: Fueling Your Afternoon:

- Lunch provides the energy you need to power through the afternoon. It should include a mix of lean proteins, whole grains, and vegetables to maintain energy levels and keep you satisfied.

4. Afternoon Snack: Beating the Slump:

- In the mid-afternoon, it's common to experience a drop in energy. A light, protein-rich snack like hummus and vegetables or a piece of fruit with peanut butter can help you stay alert.

5. Dinner: The Evening Reset:

- Dinner should be a balanced, but slightly lighter, meal compared to lunch. Include lean proteins, vegetables, and whole grains. Avoid large portions or heavy, rich foods too close to bedtime to aid digestion and promote better sleep.

6. Evening Snack: Smart Choices:

- If you feel hungry before bed, choose a light, nutritious snack like a small bowl of yogurt or a piece of whole grain toast. Avoid heavy or high-sugar options that might disrupt your sleep.

7. Hydration Throughout the Day:

- Staying adequately hydrated is crucial at all times. Include water, herbal teas, and other low-calorie beverages throughout your day. Proper hydration truly supports digestion and also the overall well-being.

8. Mindful Eating:

- Pay apt attention to your body's hunger and fullness cues always. It's advisable to eat when you're hungry, and stop when you're satisfied. Mindful eating promotes a healthy relationship with food and can help prevent overeating.

It's important to remember that meal timing can vary based on your individual schedule and preferences. The key is to ensure that you're distributing your meals and snacks throughout the day to maintain consistent energy levels and support your nutritional needs.

In the following chapters, we'll explore how to combine these meals and snacks with the seven classes of food for a balanced and healing diet tailored to your specific goals and health concerns.

CHAPTER 4

COMBINING FOODS FOR OPTIMAL HEALTH

Achieving optimal health through your diet is not just about what you eat but also about how you combine different classes of food. Proper food 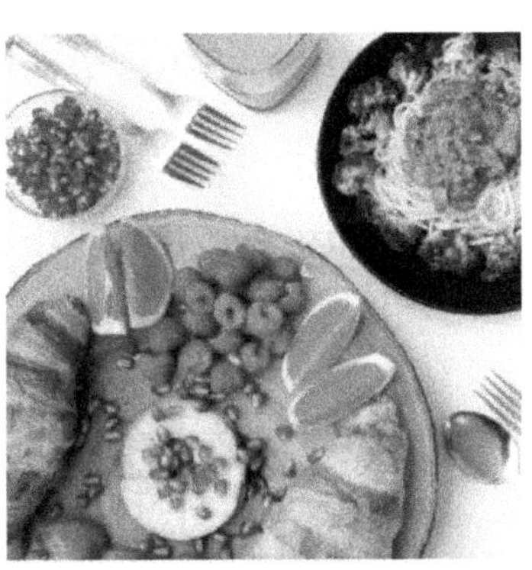 *combinations can enhance nutrient absorption, support digestion, and promote overall well-being. In this chapter, we'll delve into the art of combining foods for your health.*

1. Pairing Proteins and Carbohydrates:

- Combining lean proteins with complex carbohydrates is a winning strategy. For example, chicken breast with brown rice or beans with whole grain pasta. This balance provides both immediate and sustained energy, keeping you full and focused.

2. The Power of Fiber:

- Fiber-rich foods, such as vegetables, fruits, and whole grains, should be a part of every meal. They help regulate blood sugar, aid digestion, and provide a feeling of fullness. A salad with mixed greens, colorful vegetables, and beans is an excellent example.

3. The Healthy Fats Approach:

- Healthy fats like avocados, nuts, and olive oil are best paired with vegetables or whole grains. The fats help with the absorption of fat-soluble vitamins and promote satiety without causing excessive calorie intake.

4. Beware of Sugary and Starchy Combinations:

- Combining simple carbohydrates (sugars) with high-starch foods can lead to rapid spikes and crashes in blood sugar. This combination should be minimized. For instance, avoid sweetened cereals with added sugar.

5. Protein Diversity:

- A variety of protein sources should be incorporated into your diet. Combining plant-based proteins, such as beans, lentils, and tofu, with animal proteins diversifies your amino acid intake, promoting overall health.

6. Eating with the Seasons:

- Consider the seasonality of foods. Eating locally and seasonally can lead to more balanced nutrition, as nature provides what our bodies need at different times of the year.

7. Hydration and Timing:

- Stay hydrated, but avoid drinking large quantities of water during meals. Drinking water before or between meals supports digestion. Overloading on fluids during meals can dilute digestive juices.

8. Mindful Eating:

- Ensure to practice mindful eating by savoring your food, chewing slowly, and also paying attention to your body's hunger and fullness cues. This mindful approach enhances digestion and ensures you're eating for nourishment.

The art of combining foods is a skill that can be learned and adapted to your specific dietary preferences and health goals. Proper food combinations can lead to better digestion, increased nutrient absorption, and overall improved health. In the upcoming chapters, we'll explore specific meal plans and recipes that incorporate these principles for a balanced and healing diet.

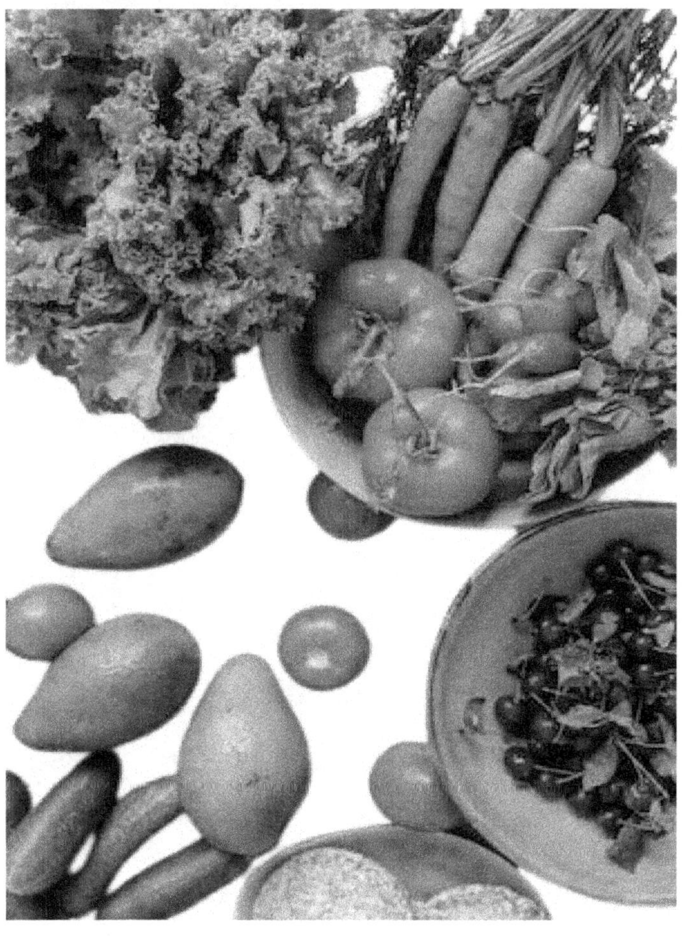

CHAPTER 5

Maintaining a healthy and healing diet isn't just about what you should eat, but also about what to avoid. As we age, it becomes even 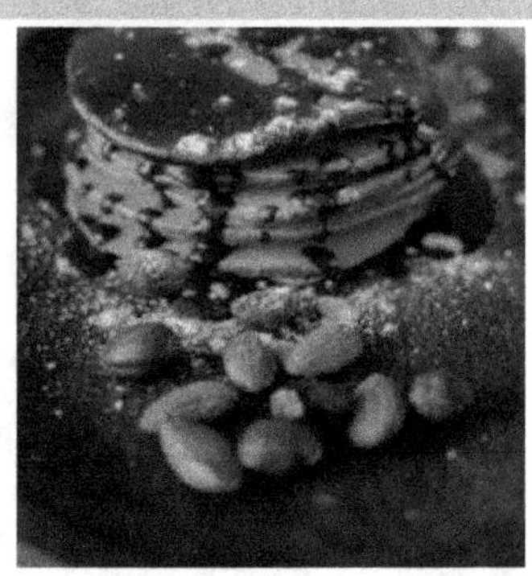 *more crucial to make informed choices to support our well-being. In this chapter, we'll identify foods and eating habits that you should steer clear of, especially as you age.*

1. Excess Sugar:

- Consuming high amounts of added sugars, often found in sodas, candies, and many processed foods, can contribute to weight gain, type 2 diabetes, and heart problems. Limit your intake of sugary treats.

2. Processed and Fast Foods:

- Highly processed and fast foods are often high in unhealthy trans fats, sodium, and empty calories. They can lead to weight gain and various health issues. Choose whole, unprocessed foods whenever possible.

3. High-Sodium Foods:

- Excessive sodium intake, typically found in canned soups, processed meats, and many restaurant dishes, can lead to hypertension and other cardiovascular problems. Choose low-sodium options and use herbs and spices for flavoring instead.

4. Trans Fats:

- Trans fats, often listed as "partially hydrogenated oils" in ingredient lists, are harmful for heart health. These fats are commonly found in fried and packaged foods. Check labels and avoid products with trans fats.

5. Large, Heavy Meals Before Bed:

- Eating substantial meals too close to bedtime can disrupt sleep and lead to indigestion. Aim for lighter evening meals that promote restful sleep.

6. Excessive Alcohol:

- While moderate alcohol consumption may have some health benefits, excessive alcohol intake can lead to a range of health problems, including liver damage and an increased risk of accidents. Keep alcohol consumption within recommended limits.

7. Empty-Calorie Snacking:

- Snacking on foods with little nutritional value, like potato chips or sugary snacks, can lead to excessive calorie intake without providing essential nutrients.

Choose healthier snack options like nuts, fruits, or yogurt.

8. Overly Restrictive Diets:

- Nutrient deficiencies and other health issues can be caused by extreme dieting or overly restrictive eating habits . Instead, focus on balanced, sustainable dietary choices.

9. Unhealthy Cooking Methods:

- Avoid frying or deep-frying foods in unhealthy oils, as these cooking methods can increase the calorie and trans fat content of your meals. Consider choosing healthier cooking methods like baking, grilling, or steaming.

10. Ignoring Dietary Allergies and Sensitivities:

- As you age, you may develop food allergies or sensitivities. Ignoring these can lead to discomfort and health issues.

Importantly, pay attention to how your body reacts to certain foods and adjust your diet accordingly.

This chapter highlights foods and habits that are best avoided to maintain and improve your health, particularly as you age. It's essential to make informed choices about what you eat and how you eat it to support your well-being.

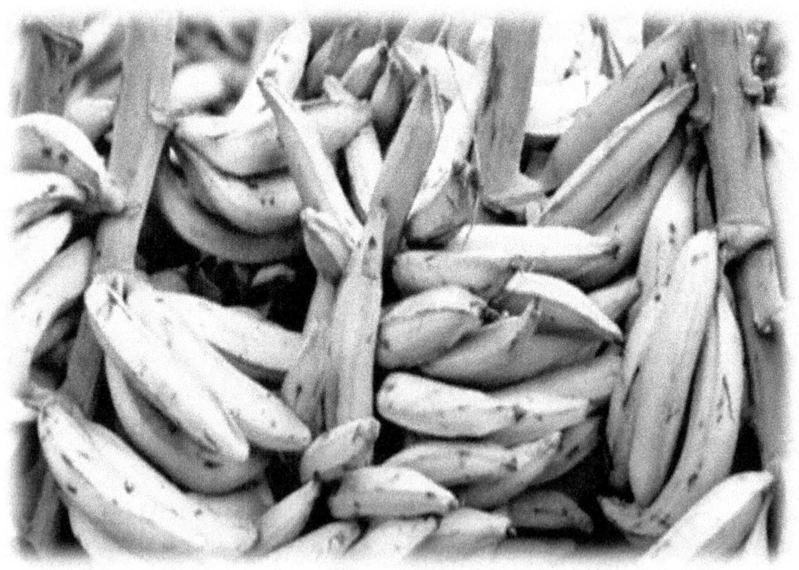

CHAPTER 6

TAILORING YOUR DIET TO YOUR AGE

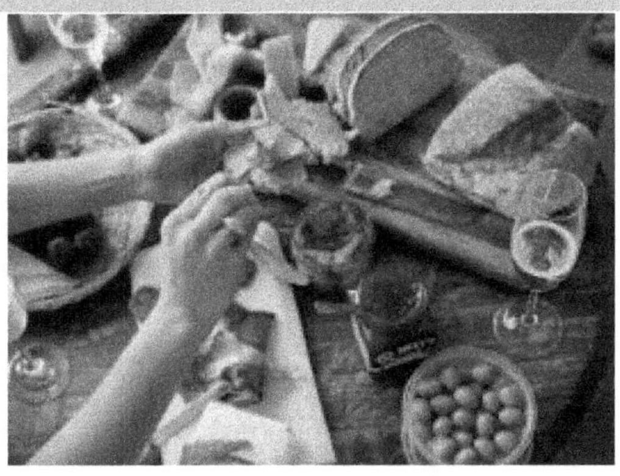

As we journey through life, our nutritional needs evolve. Age plays a significant role in determining how our bodies process and utilize nutrients. In this chapter, we'll explore how to adapt your diet to match the unique requirements of various life stages, ensuring you age gracefully and healthily.

1. Childhood and Adolescence: Building Strong Foundations:

- During these critical years, the focus should be on a balanced diet that supports growth, development, and strong bones. Nutrient-dense foods, including calcium-rich dairy products, lean proteins, whole grains, and plenty of fruits and vegetables, are essential.

2. Young Adulthood: Nutritional Variety and Fitness:

- This is a period of establishing healthy habits. Prioritize diverse food choices, exercise, and staying well-hydrated. It's also an ideal time to adopt a diet that reduces the risk of chronic diseases later in life.

3. Adulthood: Meeting the Daily Demands:

- As you age, your metabolism may slow down. Focus on portion control and nutrient-dense foods, emphasizing fiber, lean proteins, and healthy fats. Adequate calcium intake remains essential to support bone health.

4. Pregnancy and Lactation: Special Nutritional Needs:

- During pregnancy and breastfeeding, you require additional nutrients. Ensure you get sufficient folic acid, iron, and calcium. Ensure to consult with a healthcare provider to help you tailor your diet to your specific needs.

5. Middle Age: Hormonal Changes and Weight Management:

- As hormonal changes occur, maintaining a healthy weight becomes more challenging. Prioritize foods that support hormonal balance, such as whole grains, lean proteins, and foods rich in phytoestrogens. Pay attention to heart health by limiting saturated fats and salt.

6. The Golden Years: Nutrient-Rich and Fiber-Focused:

- As you enter your senior years, focus on nutrient-dense foods and high-fiber options. Adequate protein intake remains vital to preserve muscle mass. Be mindful of hydration and consider dietary supplements if necessary, especially for vitamin B12.

7. Managing Chronic Conditions: Customized Nutrition:

- If you have specific health conditions, such as diabetes, heart disease, or digestive issues, work closely with a healthcare provider or nutritionist to tailor your diet to your unique needs. Specialized dietary plans can help manage and alleviate these conditions.

8. Hydration: A Lifelong Necessity:

- Adequate hydration is crucial at every age. As you get older, your sense of thirst may diminish, making it essential to consciously drink water and consume hydrating foods like fruits and vegetables.

Incorporating these age-appropriate dietary guidelines into your life ensures that your nutrition aligns with the demands of each life stage. Remember, it's never too late to adopt healthy eating habits, and the right diet can enhance your quality of life at any age. In the following chapters, we'll provide practical strategies and meal plans for implementing these principles in your daily life.

CHAPTER 7

PRACTICAL TIPS FOR A HEALTHIER DIET

In this chapter, we'll provide practical strategies and tips to help you implement the principles discussed throughout this book into your daily life. These strategies are designed to make it easier for you to maintain a balanced and healing diet for optimal health and well-being.

1. Meal Planning:

- Plan your meals in advance. Create a weekly meal plan that includes a variety of foods from the seven classes, and prepare a shopping list to help you stick to your healthy choices.

2. Portion Control:

- Be mindful of portion sizes to avoid overeating. Practice using smaller plates and listen to your body's hunger and fullness cues.

3. Slow and Mindful Eating:

- Chew your food slowly and savor each bite. Eating mindfully allows your body to better register fullness, preventing overconsumption.

4. Balanced Plate:

- Target a balanced plate with vegetables, lean proteins, whole grains, and healthy fats. Fill half your plate with vegetables and fruits, one-quarter with lean proteins, and one-quarter with whole grains.

5. Snack Smart:

- Choose healthy snacks such as yogurt, nuts, or fruits when you need a quick energy boost. Avoid sugary and high-sodium snacks.

6. Stay Hydrated:

- Keep a reusable water bottle with you to remind yourself to drink enough water throughout the day. Hydration is essential for overall health.

7. Variety is Key:

- Explore different foods from the seven classes and incorporate a wide range of fruits, vegetables, proteins, and whole grains into your diet. Variety ensures a broad spectrum of nutrients.

8. Read Food Labels:

- Always pay attention to food labels to help you make informed choices. Look for products with simple ingredients and minimal added sugars, trans fats, and sodium.

9. Cook at Home:

- Preparing meals at home gives you control over the ingredients and cooking methods. It also encourages the use of fresh, whole foods.

10. Limit Eating Out: - Dining out can be enjoyable, but restaurant meals often contain excessive calories, unhealthy fats, and large portions. Reserve eating out for special occasions.

11. Listen to Your Body: - Pay attention to how different foods make you feel. If a particular food doesn't sit well with you or causes discomfort, consider reducing or eliminating it from your diet.

12. Seek Professional Guidance: - If you have specific health concerns or dietary restrictions, consult with a registered dietitian or healthcare provider. They can provide personalized guidance and meal plans.

13. Set Realistic Goals: - Make gradual changes to your diet. Setting realistic goals and celebrating small victories can help you maintain a healthy eating pattern over the long term.

Remember that adopting a healthy and healing diet is a lifelong journey. It's not about perfection but making consistent, informed choices that support your well-being. By applying these practical tips and the principles discussed in this book, you can enhance your health and promote healing through your dietary choices.

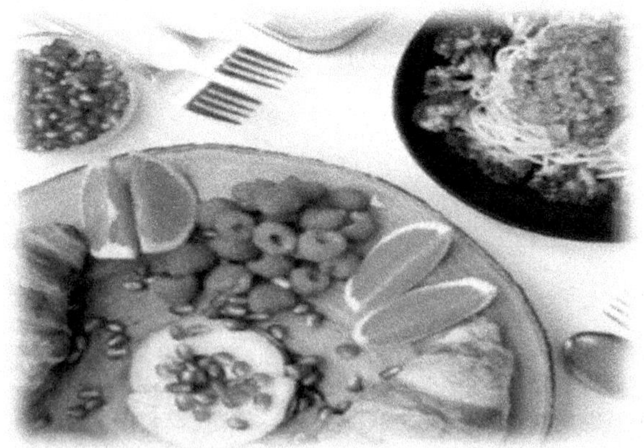

CHAPTER 8

PERSONALIZED NUTRITION PLANS AND SAMPLE MEAL PLANS

As we've journeyed through the world of nutrition, you've gained valuable insights into the importance of 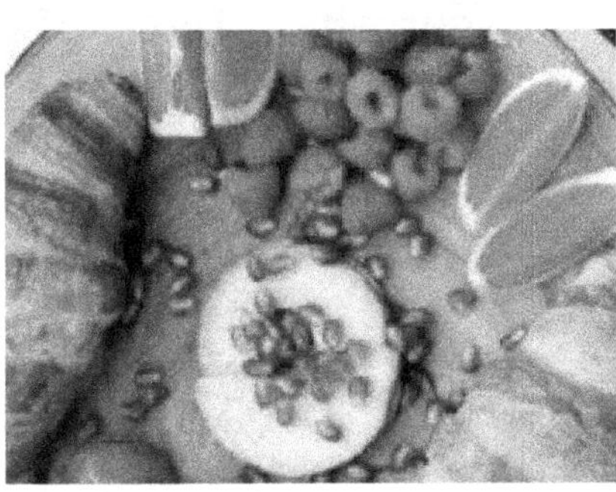 balanced eating and how to make informed choices. In this chapter, we will take the knowledge you've acquired and apply it to create personalized nutrition plans that suit your individual needs and preferences. Additionally, we'll provide a selection of sample meal plans to get you started on your path to healthier eating.

1. **Assess Your Goals:** Start by defining your nutritional goals. Are you looking to lose weight, gain muscle, manage a health condition, or simply maintain your current state of well-being? Knowing your goals will guide your plan.

2. **Determine Your Caloric Needs:** Calculate your daily caloric needs based on your goals, age, gender, activity level, and other factors. Understanding your calorie requirements is the foundation of your nutrition plan.

3. **Balancing the Seven Classes of Food:** Incorporate a variety of foods from the seven classes in appropriate proportions. For example, your plate should include lean proteins, whole grains, plenty of vegetables, and a source of healthy fats.

4. **Include Nutrient-Dense Foods:** Prioritize nutrient-dense foods like fruits, vegetables, whole grains, and lean proteins. These foods provide very important vitamins and minerals without excessive calories.

5. **Watch Your Portions:** Pay attention to portion sizes to avoid overeating. Smaller plates and also listening to your body's hunger and fullness cues can help greatly.

6. **Hydration Matters:** Ensure you consume enough water throughout the day. Proper hydration helps digestion and overall well-being.

Sample Meal Plans:

To give you a practical sense of how to apply these principles, we've created sample meal plans for different dietary goals. Keep in mind that these are just examples, and you can modify them to suit your specific preferences and requirements.

Sample Meal Plan 1: Weight Management

- Breakfast: example include Greek yogurt with mixed berries and just a sprinkle of granola.

- Snack: Carrot and cucumber sticks with hummus.

- Lunch: Grilled chicken breast with quinoa and a side of steamed broccoli.

- Snack: A small apple with a tablespoon of peanut butter.

- Dinner: Baked salmon with a side salad of mixed greens, cherry tomatoes, and olive oil dressing.

- Snack: Low-fat cottage cheese with pineapple.

Sample Meal Plan 2: Muscle Building

- Breakfast: example include oatmeal with sliced bananas and a scoop of protein powder.

- Snack: Almonds and dried apricots.

- Lunch: Turkey and avocado sandwich on whole-grain bread and also with a side of mixed greens.

- Snack: Greek yogurt with honey.

- Dinner: Lean beef stir-fry with brown rice and a variety of vegetables.

- Snack: Cottage cheese with mixed berries.

Sample Meal Plan 3: Managing a Health Condition

- Breakfast: Scrambled eggs with spinach combined with whole-grain toast.

- Snack: Sliced bell peppers with guacamole.

- Lunch: Quinoa salad with chickpeas, cucumber, and lemon-tahini dressing.

- Snack: A small orange.

- Dinner: Baked cod with asparagus together with a side of quinoa.

- Snack: A few unsalted almonds.

By creating your personalized nutrition plan and exploring sample meal plans like these, you'll be better equipped to meet your dietary goals and maintain a balanced and healing diet. Remember that your plan should be adaptable and sustainable, allowing you to enjoy a lifetime of health and well-being.

CHAPTER 9

Examples Of Food, Fruits, And Vegetables Categorized Into The Seven Classes Of Food, Along With Their Benefits And Advantages Of Eating Them In Moderation

1. Carbohydrates:

- **Foods:** Whole grains (e.g., brown rice, quinoa, whole wheat pasta)

- **Fruits:** Berries (e.g., strawberries, blueberries)

- **Vegetables:** Sweet potatoes, squash

- **Benefits:** Carbohydrates provide energy, support brain function, and are a good source of dietary fiber.

- **Advantages of Moderation:** Eating carbohydrates in moderation helps maintain stable blood sugar levels and prevents overconsumption of calories.

2. Proteins:

- **Foods:** Lean meats (e.g., chicken, turkey, lean cuts of beef)

- **Fruits:** Avocado (a source of healthy fats)

- **Vegetables:** Spinach, broccoli

- **Benefits:** Proteins are essential for tissue repair, muscle maintenance, and overall growth.

- **Advantages of Moderation:** Consuming proteins in moderation supports muscle health and satiety without excessive calorie intake.

3. Fats:

- **Foods:** Avocado, nuts (e.g., almonds, walnuts), olive oil

- **Fruits:** Olives

- **Vegetables:** Avocado, nuts, and seeds

- **Benefits:** Healthy fats support brain health, nutrient absorption, and provide a source of long-lasting energy.

- **Advantages of Moderation:** Consuming healthy fats in moderation prevents excessive calorie intake while benefiting from their nutritional value.

4. Vitamins:

- **Foods:** Citrus fruits (e.g., oranges, grapefruits), leafy greens (e.g., kale, spinach)

- **Fruits:** Kiwi, strawberries

- **Vegetables:** Bell peppers, broccoli

- **Benefits:** Vitamins play various roles in maintaining health, from supporting the immune system (e.g., vitamin C) to promoting healthy vision (e.g., vitamin A).

- **Advantages of Moderation:** Vitamins are essential, but excessive intake can be harmful. Eating them in moderation ensures a balanced intake.

5. Minerals:

- **Foods:** Dairy products (e.g., milk, yogurt), seeds (e.g., sunflower seeds), seafood (e.g., salmon, sardines)

- **Fruits:** Bananas (source of potassium)

- **Vegetables:** Spinach (rich in iron), sweet potatoes (rich in potassium)

- **Benefits:** Minerals are vital for bone health (e.g., calcium), nerve function (e.g., potassium), and blood health (e.g., iron).

- **Advantages of Moderation:** Balanced mineral intake ensures proper bodily functions, but excessive intake can lead to imbalances.

6. Fiber:

- **Foods:** Whole grains, legumes (e.g., lentils, black beans)

- **Fruits:** Apples, pears

- **Vegetables:** Broccoli, Brussels sprouts

- **Benefits:** Fiber supports digestive health, regulates blood sugar, and aids in weight management.

- **Advantages of Moderation:** While fiber is essential, excessive intake can cause digestive discomfort. It's important to consume it in balance.

7. Water:

- **Foods:** Watermelon, cucumbers (contain high water content)

- **Benefits:** Water is vital for hydration, temperature regulation, and overall bodily functions.

- **Advantages of Moderation:** Adequate hydration is essential, but overconsumption of water in a short period can lead to water intoxication.

Remember, a well-balanced diet includes a variety of foods from these categories, consumed in moderation. This approach provides the necessary nutrients for optimal health while preventing overconsumption of calories or potential nutrient imbalances.

CONCLUSION

In closing, I hope this book has shed light on the importance of nutrition in your life. Nutrition isn't just about eating; it's about making choices that impact your health and well-being every day.

Remember, small changes can lead to big improvements. Whether you aim to manage your weight, stay healthy, or simply enjoy a better life, the power of nutrition is in your hands.

Keep making informed choices about the foods you consume, stay mindful of balance and moderation, and you'll find that your journey towards health is lifelong and rewarding.

Here's to a healthier, happier you. Thank you for coming along with us on this journey.

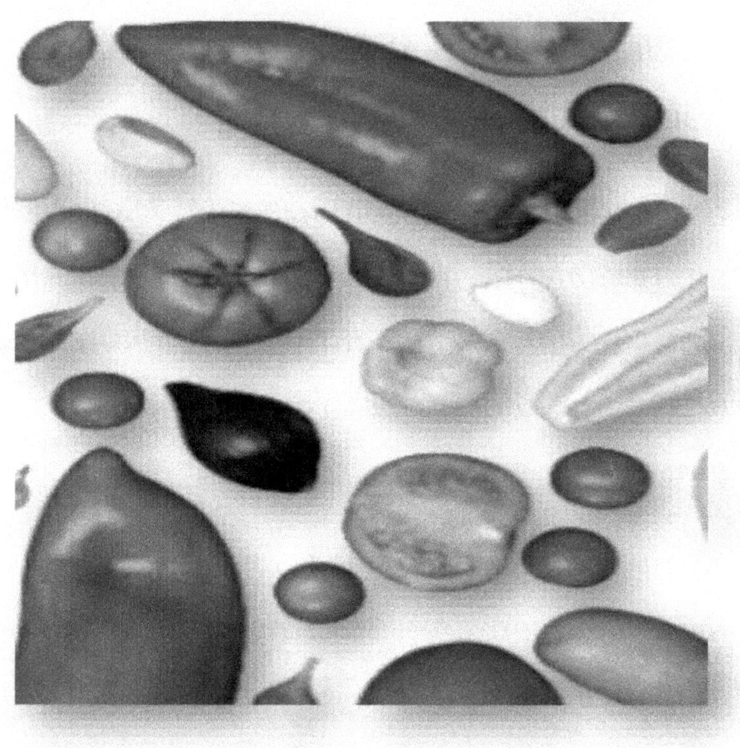

1. **Calorie:** A unit of measurement for the energy content of food. Consuming more calories than your body uses can lead to weight gain, while a calorie deficit can result in weight loss.

2. **Nutrient:** A substance in food that provides nourishment and is necessary for the body to function properly. Nutrients for example include vitamins, minerals, carbohydrates, proteins, and fats.

3. **Carbohydrate:** One of the three macronutrients, carbohydrates are the body's primary source of energy. They include sugars, starches, and fiber.

4. **Protein:** Another macronutrient, proteins are essential for tissue repair,

muscle growth, and various bodily functions. They comprise of amino acids.

5. **Fat:** A macronutrient that provides long-lasting energy, supports cell growth, and helps the body absorb fat-soluble vitamins. Healthy fats comprise of monounsaturated and polyunsaturated fats.

6. **Vitamin:** Organic compounds found in food that are essential for various physiological functions. Each vitamin has specific roles in maintaining health.

7. **Mineral:** Inorganic compounds that the body requires in small amounts to perform various functions. Common minerals include calcium, iron, and potassium.

8. **Fiber:** A type of carbohydrate found in plant foods that is not digestible by the

human body. It aids in digestion, helps maintain healthy blood sugar levels, and supports heart health.

9. **Hydration:** The process of maintaining adequate water content in the body. Proper hydration is very crucial for overall health.

10. **Portion Control:** The practice of managing the quantity of food consumed during a meal to prevent overeating and maintain a healthy calorie balance.

11. **Moderation:** Refers to the practice of consuming all types of food in appropriate and reasonable amounts, avoiding extremes in overindulgence or restriction.

12. **Nutrient-Dense:** Foods that provide a high concentration of relevant nutrients relative to their calorie content.

Nutrient-dense foods are considered healthy choices.

13.   **Whole Grains:** Grains that include the entire grain kernel, including the bran, germ, and endosperm. They are a good source of fiber, vitamins, and minerals.

14.   **Lean Proteins:** Protein sources that are low in saturated fats. Examples include skinless poultry, fish, and lean cuts of beef.

15.   **Vegetarian:** A dietary pattern that excludes meat and seafood but may include dairy products and eggs. Variations exist, such as lacto-vegetarian and ovo-vegetarian diets.

16.   **Vegan:** A diet that does not all animal products, including meat, dairy, and eggs.

17.   **Plant-Based Diet:** A diet centered around plant foods, which can include fruits, vegetables, whole grains, legumes, nuts, seeds, and spices. It may or may not exclude animal products.

18.   **Spices:** Spices are dried, aromatic, and often ground plant parts used to flavor and season food. They are derived from various parts of plants, including seeds, bark, roots, and fruits. Spices can add depth and complexity to the taste of dishes and are often used in cooking for their flavor-enhancing properties. They can be both whole (e.g., cinnamon sticks, whole peppercorns) and ground (e.g., ground cinnamon, black pepper). Spices are a vital component of culinary traditions around the world and can have health benefits beyond their culinary use due to their potential medicinal properties.

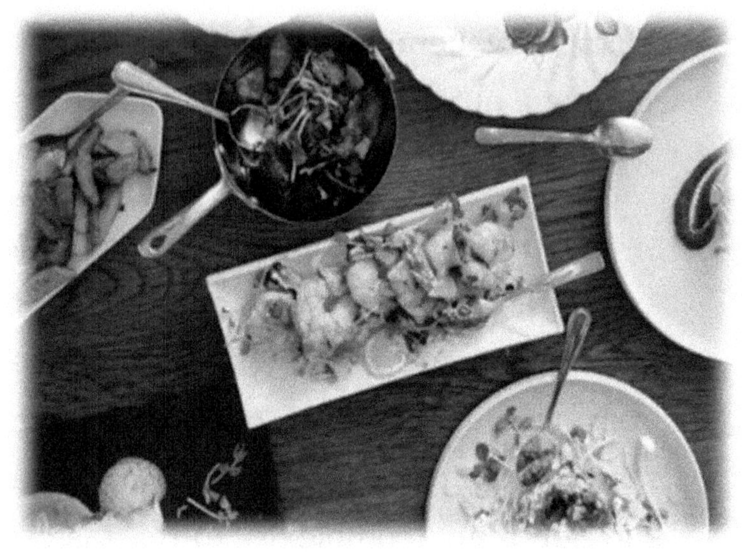

Thanks for Reading, and

Happy Healthy Living.